YOUR HEART, YOUR LIFE

Greatest Ways Of Preventing And Defeating Heart Diseases

By

Mary J. Douglas

TABLE OF CONTENTS

INTRODUCTION

The main advantage of reading "Your Heart, Your Life" is that it will serve as an inspiration for you to take action to enhance your heart health. You may have made efforts to protect your heart and lower your risk of acquiring heart disease by becoming aware of the risk factors and lifestyle modifications that can help avoid this condition. Millions of individuals worldwide are affected by the growing epidemic of heart disease. In many nations, it is the most cause of mortality, and the incidence is rising. But what if there was a method to stop it completely or reverse it? You can learn the most recent course of action and research on heart health in this ground-breaking book. This detailed manual is brimming with very useful suggestions and guidance for maintaining a heart healthy lifestyle, from food adjustments to exercise routines.

The most prevalent risk factors for heart disease, such as excessive blood pressure, high cholesterol, and smoking, will be discussed. Also, you will learn how to lower your risk by implementing easy lifestyle modifications, including eating a heart-healthy diet, exercising frequently, and stress management.

That is not all, though. Also, if you have already been diagnosed with heart disease, this book will explain how to reverse it. You will learn about the best medical interventions, surgical procedures, and lifestyle modifications.

This book is your definitive guide to a healthier heart, whether your goal is to avoid heart disease or reverse it. You will be on your road to better health in no time with these simple guidance and professional insights.

CHAPTER 1

DEFINITION OF HEART DISEASE AND ITS TYPES

Heart disease is a general term for a variety of cardiac problems. Cardiovascular ailments, which makes reference to heart and blood vessel disease, is another name for it. Coronary heart disease, which is the most prevalent kind of heart disease in the US, affects heart blood flow. A heart attack may be brought on by decreased blood flow.

The signs or symptoms of a heart attack, heart failure, or arrhythmia may not be noticed until after a person has been diagnosed with a heart illness that is "silent" or undiagnosed. In the United States, heart disease is the primary cause of mortality for both men and women, but there are strategies to prevent and treat many different types of heart conditions.The main signs of a heart attack in men and women include:

Chest discomfort or agony. Larger number of heart attacks are identified by chest pain on the left or centre sides that lasts for more than a few minutes or that fades and reappears. The discomfort may feel

like a painful pressure, squeezing, fullness, or other unpleasant sensation,
feeling flimsy, dizzy, or faint. Also, you can start to sweat a lot.
Back, neck, or jaw discomfort or pain.
One or both arms or shoulders may experience pain or discomfort.
Respiration difficulty. Shortness of breath can occur before chest discomfort, although it also frequently occurs together.
Additional heart attack symptoms may include extreme or unexpected fatigue, nausea, or vomiting.
Some other symptoms are more common in women

Heart Disease Types

Cardiovascular artery disease (CAD): The most ubiquitous type of cardiac disease in the US is coronary artery disease (CAD). It is also known as ischemic heart disease or coronary heart disease. A heart attack may be the inceptive symptom of CAD in some patients. Your capability to minimise your risk for CAD entirely depends on you and your medical team. Formation of plaques in the walls of the coronary arteries, which provide blood to the heart and other parts of the body, results in CAD. Layers of cholesterol and other materials in the artery form plaque. With time, plaque development causes the interior of the arteries to thin, which can obstruct blood flow either partially or totally. Atherosclerosis is the name of this process.

Heart Attack: When the heart muscle is not oxygenated sufficiently in one or more places, the heart muscle's blood supply is restricted, and heart attack (myocardial infarction) results.
The augmentation of plaque in the arteries is the principal cause of the blockage (atherosclerosis). Deposits of cholesterol and other materials make up plaques As soon as a plaque ruptures, a blood clot forms which induces heart attack. The Heart muscle cells start to incur damage and begin to die if the blood and oxygen supply is interrupted. During 30 minutes of interruption, irreversible harm starts. As a result, the cardiac muscle that is affected by the lack of oxygen can no longer function properly.
Heart valve disease: The mitral, tricuspid, pulmonary, and aortic are the four heart valves that maintain proper blood flow. There are paperlike flaps on each valve that open and close one after the other once every heartbeat. Blood flow from your

heart to your body is interrupted if one or more valves do not open or seal correctly. Heart valve disease can be congenitally present at birth and or develop in adults due to a variety of reasons and circumstances, including infections and other heart problems. Heart valve problems can make your heart work harder if not treated. Your quality of life can negatively be affected and even endanger your life. Your healthcare practitioner may be able to replace or repair your heart valves by surgery or minimally invasive treatment in many circumstances, restoring normal function and enabling you to resume your normal activities.

Heart arrhythmia: An erratic heartbeat is known as heart arrhythmia. When the electrical signals that control how often the heart beats do not correlate properly, heart rhythm issues (heart arrhythmias) result. The heart beats rapidly without restraints (tachycardia), too slowly (bradycardia), or irregularly as a result of poor signalling. Cardiac arrhythmias, which may be completely safe, sometimes feel like your heart is speeding or fluttering. Yet, some heart rhythms can result in unwelcome and perhaps even life-threatening symptoms. But, occasionally having a fast or sluggish heart rate is natural, for example the rate of heart may rise during physical activity or fall during sleep.

Arterial disease of the periphery: A disorder of the blood vessels that do not serve the heart or brain is known as peripheral arterial disease (PAD). A development of fatty deposits in the arteries frequently causes PAD. Peripheral vascular disease or peripheral arterial disease are other names for PAD (which includes both arteries and veins). Blood flow to the arms, kidneys, stomach, and—most frequently the legs is restricted because of PAD's effect on blood arteries, which causes them to constrict. Peripheral artery disease, which affects 12 to 20 percent of Americans over 60, is thought to afflict 8.5 million people in the US. A significant risk factor for heart attack and stroke is peripheral arterial disease. In comparison to women, men are slightly more prone to acquire PAD. Smokers also tend to have peripheral vascular disease more frequently.

Cardiomyopathy: Cardiomyopathy is a term used to describe different diseases of the heart muscle in which the walls of the heart chambers have become stretched, thickened, stiffened, thinned out, or filled with substances the body produces that are not supposed to be in the heart muscle. As a result, the heart muscle's ability to pump blood reduces and can cause irregular heartbeats, diminishes flow of blood into the lungs or the rest of the body, and heart failure. These illnesses can affect people of various ages and races. Majority of hereditary forms of cardiomyopathy affect youngsters and younger people. Cardiomyopathy can be inherited or caused by another ailment.

Congenital heart disease: The heart eventually becomes too weak or stiff to fill and pump blood correctly due to several heart disorders, such as coronary artery disease (narrowing of the heart's arteries) or high blood pressure.

Around 6 million Americans suffer from heart failure. Heart failure is confirmed in about 670,000 persons annually. It is the predominant cause of hospital admission for individuals over 65.

Heart failure does not signify the stoppage of the heart beat but rather, the heart has weakened and doesn't work to perfection. Blood pressure in the heart rises and blood flow through the heart and body slows down due to a number of potential causes. As a result, the heart is incapable of pumping the body's requirements for oxygen and nourishment.

The heart's chambers may react by expanding to accommodate more blood to pump through the body or by stiffening and thickening to keep the blood flowing but with time, the muscle walls may deteriorate and lose their ability to pump as effectively as possible. The body may begin to retain fluid (water) and salt because of the kidneys' reaction. The body becomes clogged if fluid accumulates in the limbs, legs, ankles, feet, lungs, or other organs. This condition is known as congestive heart disease.

Aortic aneurysm: The aorta is a very large artery in the human body. It conveys oxygen enriched blood from your heart to the rest of your body. It has a curled candy cane form. Your heart's aorta ascends from there. The cavity within your abdomen is reached by means of your descending aorta (belly). Aortic aneurysm can attack any of the arteries. When the strength of your aorta wall diminishes, an aortic aneurysm can form. The weak spot of your aorta develops a balloon-like protrusion due to the pressure of blood pumping through the artery. Aortic aneurysm is the name given to this protrusion. Aortic aneurysms may split open or burst:

Segregation of the arterial wall's layers may occur due to the stress of blood pumping, causing blood to seep in between them. This course of action is known as a dissection.

Aneurysms have the potential to burst entirely, resulting in internal bleeding, also known as rupture. Most aortic aneurysm deaths are influenced by dissections and ruptures. The two forms of aortic aneurysms are different. They impact several body parts, including:

Aortic aneurysm of the abdomen (AAA): An abdominal aortic aneurysm is formed in the downward-pointing "handle" of your aorta.

A thoracic aortic aneurysm (TAA) is a heart aneurysm that develops in the area of your aorta that is shaped like an upside-down U. A TAA in the ascending aorta can happen in persons with Marfan syndrome, a condition affecting the connective tissues.

Myocarditis: The most frequent cause of myocarditis, or heart muscle inflammation, is a viral infection (myocardium). The heart's ability to pump blood is weakened by this uncommon heart ailment. People may experience this illness suddenly or gradually over time. While some people do not exhibit any symptoms, others do. Myocarditis is often treated with medications.

Myocarditis differs from other forms of inflammation since they all affect various areas of the heart. Your heart's surrounding sac is impacted by pericarditis. An infection or inflammation of your heart valves is known as endocarditis.

Individuals who have myocarditis frequently experience exhaustion, shortness of breath, chest pain, or a racing heart (palpitations). People might experience these symptoms slowly over time or they might experience them suddenly. Advanced myocarditis patients may experience heart failure symptoms.

CHAPTER 2

UNDERSTANDING THE FUNDAMENTALS OF HEART HEALTH

The circulatory system is a web of arteries and veins that the heart, a muscular organ the size of a fist, pumps blood through. It is situated behind and somewhat to the left of the breastbone. It is the main organ of your circulatory system. The heart is divided into four primary muscle-powered chambers. The nervous system and brain control how your heart beats.

The heart is crucial to how the human body works.

- Its important function is to circulate blood throughout the body.
- Makes it possible for the blood to be transported with oxygen to every part of the body.
- Assists in maintaining adequate blood pressure throughout the body.

- Delivers nutrients to all the body's cells, tissues, and organs.

Living a heart-healthy lifestyle means being aware of your risk factors, making positive decisions, and taking actions to lower your risk of developing heart disease, including the most prevalent type, coronary heart disease. You can reduce your risk of getting heart disease, which could cause a heart attack, by practising preventive methods.

5 Strategies For A Healthy Heart

1. Take aspirin following your doctor's instructions: See a medical expert to know if taking aspirin will lessen your chance of suffering a heart attack or stroke. Tell your doctor about your medical history and any family members who have suffered from heart disease or stroke.

2. Managing your blood pressure: The amount of pressure that the blood exerts on the artery walls is measured by blood pressure. You may experience high blood pressure if your blood pressure levels are consistently high. This is known as hypertension. Compared to other risk factors, high blood pressure makes you more likely to experience a heart attack or stroke. Learn your blood pressure readings, then inquire with a medical expert about what they mean for your health. Work with a medical professional to reduce your blood pressure if you have high blood pressure.

3. Control your cholesterol levels: A waxy substance called cholesterol is produced by the liver and is present in some meals. Although your body requires cholesterol, having too much might cause heart disease by causing artery buildup. There are various types of cholesterol; one type is "good" and can reduce your risk of heart disease, while another type is "bad" and can increase it. Discuss cholesterol with your healthcare provider, including strategies to reduce excessive levels of bad cholesterol.

4. Give up smoking: Smoking causes blood pressure to rise, which boosts your risk of heart attack and stroke. Quit smoking, if you do, and discuss with your healthcare provider on how you can stick with your decision to quit.

5. Get moving: To be energetic and mobile is the main solution for having a healthy heart. It is one of your best weapons for protecting your arteries from damage caused by excessive cholesterol, high blood sugar, and high blood pressure that can cause a heart failure or stroke. It also helps to build up your heart muscles and manage your weight.

CHAPTER 3

AGENTS OF RISK FOR HEART DISEASE

Elevated blood pressure, high levels of LDL cholesterol, diabetes, smoking, exposure to secondhand smoke, obesity, a poor diet, and inactivity are the main risk factors for heart disease and stroke.

High Blood Pressure

When your blood pressure in your circulatory system is higher than usual, it is referred to as high blood pressure or hypertension. Your daily routine influences your blood pressure changes throughout the day. Systolic blood pressure over diastolic blood pressure is used to measure blood pressure. Systolic blood pressure measures the force your blood applies to the artery walls while your heart beats and diastolic blood pressure shows the amount of force your blood is applying to the walls of your arteries when your heart is at rest between beats. A systolic measurement of less than 120 mmHg and a diastolic value of less than 80 mmHg are considered to be normal blood pressure. Although high systolic or diastolic blood pressure alone can be used to diagnose high blood pressure or hypertension, elevated systolic or diastolic blood pressure is typically given greater attention to as a risk factor for cardiovascular disease. The only method to determine if you have high blood pressure, which is also very common and typically has no symptoms, is to have your blood pressure measured. Your health can detoriate by high blood pressure in many ways by severly damaging your organs like your heart, brain, kidneys, and eyes. Your arteries may become less elastic as a result of high blood pressure, which can cause damage to them and result in heart disease by reducing the amount of blood and oxygen reaching your heart. Moreover, chest pain, heart attacks, and heart failure can all occur by the reduction of blood flow to the heart.

Low Density Lipoprotein(LDL)

Low-density lipoprotein is known by the acronym LDL. It is a specific lipoprotein subtype that is present in blood. A lipid (fat) is carried through the bloodstream by lipoproteins, which are protein and lipid-based particles. Fats can not flow through your blood on their own because of the way they are structured. In order to transport fat to different cells throughout your body, lipoproteins act as transporters. Smaller amounts of proteins and a lot of cholesterol make up LDL particles. The terms "LDL" and "LDL cholesterol" are frequently used interchangeably. The expression "bad cholesterol" is used for LDL cholesterol. But that only tells a portion of the tale. LDL cholesterol is not harmful due to the crucial roles played by cholesterol in your body. Yet, difficulties can arise when your LDL cholesterol level is excessive. High LDL cholesterol makes your arteries more prone to developing plaque (atherosclerosis). The development of plaque may result in coronary artery disease.

Alzheimer's disease.

Disease of the peripheral arteries.

The aortic aneurysm.

For this reason, medical professionals advise you to maintain a healthy level of LDL cholesterol.

What is the standard level for LDL cholesterol?

The majority of adults should maintain LDL levels below 100 mg/dL. Your LDL should be lower and must be under 70 mg/dl if you have a history of atherosclerosis.

LDL level above 100 mg/dL elevates your risk of cardiovascular disease. This is how medical

professionals characterise and categorise your LDL
cholesterol level:
Normal: Below 100 mg/dL.
Ideal range: 100 to 129 mg/dL
High-risk range: 130 to 159 mg/dL.
Exceptionally high: 190 mg/dL or higher. Taking a
routine blood test, known as a lipid panel, will
determine your cholesterol levels. It is advisable to
discuss the importance of your cholesterol numbers
with your doctor as soon as you receive your
findings.

Diabetes

Diabetes mellitus is a metabolic disorder that
generates excessive glucose. It's Either your body
can not effectively use the insulin it produces or it
can not produce enough of it. Insulin is a hormone
that transports blood sugar into your cells, where it
can be stored or used as fuel. If this procedure fails
to take place in your body, you can have diabetes.
Diabetes-related high blood sugar, when left
untreated, can impair your kidneys, nerves, eyes,
and other organs. Yet, you can help protect your
welfare by having knowledge about diabetes and
taking the necessary steps to prevent or control it.
Type 1 and Type 2 diabetes are the two subtypes

that exist. Raised glucose levels are the cause of diabetes side symptoms.

High blood sugar levels over an extended length of time can harm your blood vessels if you have diabetes. Sometimes, this might result in heart attacks and strokes. Long-term kidney impairment from diabetes might make it more difficult for you to eliminate extra fluid and waste from your body. Diabetes generally has the following negative effects:

- Severe hunger
- Severe thirst
- Reduction in weight
- Continual urination
- Cloudy vision
- Too much fatigue
- Injuries that do not mend.

Exposure To Handed-Down Cigarette Smoke And Smoking

Your blood pressure briefly rises with each cigarette you smoke. Smoking damages the vein walls, which leads to atherosclerosis, a condition in which fat deposits in the walls of your arteries cause them to narrow. Moreover, it forces your blood to coagulate and strains your heart. Coronary events and strokes may result from these procedures. Smoking has a significant negative impact on your lungs, stomach, mouth, throat, and skin, producing carcinogenic growth and premature ageing. It might be detrimental to your bones and reproductive system. Regardless of how long you have smoked, giving up has immediate positive health effects. You will reduce your risk of becoming sick, breathe more effectively, and feel better overall, furthermore offer the choice of superior tasting. Those who are not smokers and engage in passive smoking, often known as handed-down smoking, which involves breathing in tobacco smoke exhaled by smokers. People in that vicinity who breath in tobacco smoke when it enters the environment are more at risk because the cigarette smoke which is handed down has already been contaminated by the smoker and the fact that you are now contaminating yourself by inhaling it makes your situation even worse. Exposure to secondhand smoke can result in a number of illnesses, including heart disease, stroke, cellular damage to the lungs as well as sudden death. It can also have negative effects on women's conceptional health, such as low birth weight.

Overweight

Obesity-Related Problems negatively impact the body and the mind. In any case, weight is the one "component" of the body which is most closely related to the others. A healthy weight allows the bones, muscles, mind, heart, and other organs to function normally and effectively for a very long period. When a person weighs more than is healthy for his or her height, this condition is referred to as obesity. It raises the risk of a number of fatal and disabling conditions, such as diabetes, heart disease, and several malignancies. Weight gain can be caused by eating habits, physical activity levels, sleep schedules, genetics, and being on some specific drugs. Obesity reduces life expectancy and quality of life while also raising personal, societal and healthcare expenses. The encouraging news is that shedding weight can limit several hazards associated with obesity. Reducing as little as 5 to 10 percent of body weight delivers considerable health benefits to those who are obese, even if they never hit their "ideal" weight, and even if they only reduce weight later in life.

Family Background

A family health history is a list of the illnesses and medical issues that members of your family have experienced. Understanding health risks and preventing diseases can be done with the help of family medical history. Studies have shown there is a chance that children and grandchildren will have hypertension if their biological parents or grandparents do. The greatest risk is when family members begin to get hypertension before the age of 55. Yet this is unaffected by lifestyle elements like exercise, drinking, and a salt-rich diet. Up to 30 to 50% of the variation in blood pressure readings in twins and families, may be explained by family history. It appears that genes contribute to hypertension, and relatives can pass these genetic features down to future generations. Yet, hereditary hypertension is caused by a combination of factors, not just genes. Another factor is that people who share living spaces may consume the same unhealthy diet or practise similar behaviours, like smoking or binge drinking. These elements, along with heredity, raise the risk of hypertension. If you have a history of hypertension in their family, they should be aware of the risk factors and try to minimise them whenever feasible.

CHAPTER 4

LIFESTYLE CHANGES FOR GOOD HEART HEALTH

Lifestyle changes are behaviour adjustments or habits modifications that promote constructive life. They are a crucial part of any wellness journey. Bad lifestyle habits include:

Eating Propensities: Unhealthy eating habits do not give your body the right kinds and amounts of nutrients it needs for optimum health. The typical American diet is overly high in calories and lacking in fruits and vegetables. Moreover, some foods are more likely to result in medical issues than others. Improper food is one of the main risk factors for several chronic diseases, including cancer, diabetes, cardiovascular disorders, and other diseases associated with obesity. Increase your intake of fruit, vegetables, legumes, nuts, and grains, according to specific dietary recommendations. Choosing unsaturated fats over saturated fats is also a good idea. Enhance your eating habits by consuming fewer salt and sugar and more fruits, vegetables, legumes, nuts, and grains.

Drinking Patterns: Water intake should be adequate because it benefits your heart as well as your brain, mood, and body weight. Dehydration and heart rate have a direct relationship. Around 2,000 litres of blood are pumped out of your body each day by your beating heart. Maintaining proper hydration, or drinking more water than you are losing, will support the work of your heart. Your body's muscles can function even better when your heart can pump blood more freely. Your heart has to work harder if you are dehydrated. When you are dehydrated, your blood volume, or the amount of blood flowing through your body, drops. Your heart beats more quickly as a result, raising your heart rate and bringing on palpitations. Moreover, more sodium is retained in your blood, making it more difficult for it to circulate throughout your body. So how much water should you consume each day to stay hydrated? It depends on how much your body needs it. You should drink extra water

If you are exercising or engaging in other physical activity,

If you suffer from a medical issue like diabetes or heart disease.

If you are exhibiting symptoms of dehydration,
such as weakness or vertigo.
Please remember that some medical problems, such
as heart failure, may call for other hydration
techniques, so consult your doctor as necessary.

Being inactive physically: Those who do not engage
in the appropriate amount of regular physical
activity are known as physically inactive. To
improve cardiovascular fitness, the American Heart
Association suggests engaging in aerobic activity for
30 to 60 minutes three to four times per week. Even
those without any additional risk factors can develop
heart disease from a lack of physical activity.
Obesity, high blood pressure, high blood cholesterol,
and type 2 diabetes are additional heart disease risks
that can arise with being obese. A variety of
exercises is indeed required to achieve whole
fitness. Although flexibility does not directly affect
heart health, it is still significant because it lays a
solid foundation for the more efficient performance
of aerobic and strength exercises. "Aerobic exercise
and resistance training are the most important for
heart health."
Here are some ways that various forms of exercise
might be beneficial to you:

Aerobic exercise: Aerobic exercise enhances circulation, which as a result lowers blood pressure. Also, it improves your cardiac output and general aerobic fitness, as shown by a treadmill test, for instance (how well your heart pumps). Moreover, aerobic activity lowers the incidence of type 2 diabetes and, if you already have the disease, aids in blood glucose control. Ideally, at least five days per week for at least 30 minutes. Running, taking a swim, riding a bicycle, playing tennis, and jumping rope are a few examples of vigorous exercise. When doctors advise at least 150 minutes per week of moderate activity, they typically mean vigorous aerobic exercise.

Strength training: This is also known as resistance training and has a more focused impact on body composition. For those who have excess body fat (including a large belly, which is a risk factor for heart disease), resistance training can help reduce fat and build lean muscle mass. According to research carried out, merging weight training with aerobic exercise may help increase HDL (good) cholesterol and decrease LDL (bad) cholesterol. Exercising with free weights (such as hand weights, dumbbells, or barbells), on a weight machine, with resistance bands, or by performing body-weight exercises like pushups, squats, and chin-ups.

Sleeping Habits: Some of the most current studies on sleep and heart health suggest that the heart prefers regular sleep. According to a study that followed older persons for five years, those with the most erratic sleep cycles had almost double the risk of developing heart disease. Researchers discovered that individuals between the ages of 45 and 84 who have irregular sleep patterns varying the timing and quantity of sleep had a higher risk of cardiovascular disease. Having a regular sleep routine may help avoid heart disease. It is critical to get adequate sleep for optimum health. Most individuals should obtain seven to nine hours of good sleep every night, according to experts. Healthy brain function as well as other components of our metabolism, such as controlling hunger and blood sugar, are supported by sleep. Lack of sleep has been linked in studies to diseases like diabetes and obesity.

Changing these behaviours can have a long-term impact on your well-being. Your weight, the health of your hormones, and the intensity of your pain can all be influenced by how much sleep you get.

How To Transform Your Lifestyle For The Better

Developing good habits takes repetition and consistency. A new activity usually feels natural after around 21 days of doing it. This implies that it would not take long for you to develop a good habit. The best approach for modifying your lifestyle is to replace bad habits with good ones. Choose a behaviour that needs to be improved and replace it with something similar rather than merely quitting a bad habit or starting a good one. Simple hand-weight exercises or jogging on a treadmill while watching TV, for instance, can replace the habit of nibbling while watching TV. Changes in lifestyle fall into three main kinds. They are as follows: Psychological, behavioural , and dietary changes. Emotional and stress management are all examples of psychological changes. Join a support group or keep a journal as the tool to help you go through healthy psychological changes.

Changes in behaviour include factors like your sleeping patterns, level of activity, managing your time and planning attempts,

Changes to your nutrition: Losing weight, balancing hormone levels, and managing pain can all be achieved with a balanced diet. Controlling portion sizes, consuming more water, and eating a balanced diet are a few of these modifications. Starting small is the best strategy for implementing long-lasting improvements in your life. This requires looking at each habit you have and assessing how it affects your way of living. When necessary, make straightforward, practical improvements. In contrast to trying to fully restructure your existing way of life, changing just one behavior at a time can result in long-lasting changes in your life.

CHAPTER 5

MEDICATIONS AND SURGERIES FOR HEART DISEASE TREATMENT

Blood Thinners

Anticoagulants, also known as blood thinners, work to stop the formation of blood clots. They do not dissolve existing blood clots. They can, however, prevent such clots from growing larger. Because blood clots in your blood arteries and heart can result in heart attacks, strokes, and blockages, it is crucial to treat them.

You may need a blood thinner if you have certain blood vessel or heart conditions like:

- Atrial fibrillation
- Replacement of heart valve
- Blood clot risk following surgery
- Birth malformations of the heart

What adverse effects can blood thinners cause?

The most typical adverse reaction to blood thinners is bleeding. Moreover, they may result in diarrhoea, nausea, and upset stomach.

Depending on the type of blood thinner you are taking, additional side effects may also occur.

If you experience any symptoms of severe bleeding, such as:

- Heavy unusual menstrual flow
- Brown coloured urine
- Reddish- or black-coloured bowel movement
- bleeding from the nose or gums that do not stop right away
- Brown or vibrantly coloured vomit
- Severe discomforts, such as a migraine or stomach ache
- Strange bruising
- Bleeding from a cut that will not cease
- Dizziness

Statins

A group of medications known as statins are used to decrease cholesterol. Most of the cholesterol in your blood is produced by the liver, but some of it is derived from your diet. Statins function by assisting the liver in removing cholesterol from the blood and lowering the amount of cholesterol the liver produces. Moreover, statins might lessen arterial wall inflammation. Blockages resulting from this can harm organs including the heart and brain.

When taken as prescribed, statins can significantly lower a person's chance of having a heart attack or stroke, yet millions of individuals are not taking advantage of this benefit. Due to worries about adverse effects, people frequently discontinue taking statins or do not begin taking them. The good news is that knowing your specific advantages and dangers and discussing your worries with your clinician can help you avoid heart attacks and strokes and live a longer, healthier life.

Advantages of statins: Statins have been scientifically shown to lower a person's risk of having a heart attack, stroke, needing surgery, angioplasty, or stenting to improve blood flow in an artery, and passing away from a heart attack when used as prescribed. The statin's benefits increase in proportion to an individual's risk of suffering a heart attack or stroke. The advantage grows the longer statin is used. Generally speaking, taking statin can reduce a person's chance of having a heart attack or stroke by 50%.

Disadvantages of statins: Major dangers are uncommon. There are no differences between statin users and those taking an inactive pill, according to studies involving thousands of participants, in terms of heart related issues or muscle aches.

Notwithstanding these results, slightly over one in four (29%) statin users report experiencing some side effects, the most prevalent of which are muscle pain or weakness. It is crucial to remember that persons who are active and not taking statins frequently experience muscle-related problems with aging. In addition to muscle damage that is typically detectable with a blood test, statins have very infrequent side effects including elevated blood sugar levels or new-onset diabetes in people who are predisposed to the disease. The substantial benefit of taking statins to prevent heart attacks and strokes likely surpasses the negligible danger brought on by having high blood sugar.

Statin side effects are usually treated with dose modifications or by switching to a different statin medication. Please address your worries with your clinician so they can help you evaluate whether it is likely your symptoms are caused by the statin before quitting or changing your medication.

Beta-Blockers

A class of drugs known as beta-blockers is most frequently used for heart and circulatory system issues. To control things like blood pressure, heart rate, and more. Beta-blockers function by slowing down specific types of cell activities.

To regulate specific bodily activities and processes, your body uses a chemical signalling system, this makes use of particular cell surface locations known as receptors, where certain chemicals known as neurotransmitters can attach.

Receptors operate like locks. A molecule that has the correct structure can latch onto a receptor and act as a key to trigger the cell to respond in a particular way. Depending on its location and actions, a cell will react in a particular way. Your body can make more of the chemical that can activate the cells' receptors if certain cells are required for action. Several drugs function by tampering with that chemical signalling mechanism. Two types of medications function in this manner:

These drugs bind to and stimulate receptor sites. They effectively play the part of the appropriate chemical substance, and the cell is duped. Cells that would not otherwise be active may be stimulated by this.

These drugs bind to the receptor sites but do not affect the body in any other way. The result is comparable to when a key breaks after being inserted into a lock. Another key cannot enter because of the fractured portion of the key, which remains in place. The number of accessible receptors is decreased by antagonists, which slows down cell activity.

Beta receptors

Adrenergic receptors, also known as adrenoceptors, are an important class of receptors that are distributed all over your body. Its name comes from the neurotransmitter epinephrine, often known as adrenaline, which is created by your body.

Adrenaline can open all adrenergic receptors, much like a master key can open all the locks of a building.

Beta-blockers oppose beta-receptor, they hinder beta-adrenergic receptors and reduce particular cell activities.

Depending on where they are located, the three main subtypes of beta receptors perform various tasks.

Beta-1

The heart and kidneys are the principal locations of beta-1 receptors. They perform the following when turned on:

- Your heartbeat will quicken.

The heart's ability to pump blood Increases.

- Activate the kidney-found enzyme renin's production.

Beta-2

Beta-2 receptors are primarily present in smooth muscle tissues. The tissue is found in your blood vessels, neurological system, and respiratory system (particularly your trachea and bronchial tubes). These receptors influence numerous bodily systems in the following ways when activated:

- Cause the smooth muscles of the respiratory system to relax and make breathing easier.
- Blood vessels: Decrease blood pressure by causing the smooth muscle to relax.   Start the liver's process of converting glycogen into glucose (which your body uses for energy).
- Boost heart rate and pumping power.
- Muscle trembling is brought on by the nervous system.

Beta-3

Most fat cells and your bladder contain beta-3 receptors. They perform the following when turned on:

- Cause the decomposition of fat cells.
- Relax the body and boost bladder capacity.

- Limits the potential medical usefulness of drugs that target the B3 receptor by causing tremors.
- The following conditions, among others, are primarily treated with beta-blockers for the heart and circulatory systems:
- Rupture of the aorta.
- Arrhythmia
- Pain in the chest (angina).   Arterial disease in the heart.
- A heart attack.
- Failing heart (especially chronic heart failure).
- Excessive blood pressure (hypertension).
- Cardiomyopathy with hypertrophy and obstruction (enlarged heart).
- Migraines
- A high blood pressure in the portal veins

Benefits and risks

Benefits: They are very beneficial for a variety of medical issues. Because there are so many interconnected heart and circulation issues, treating one issue with a beta-blocker can frequently help with other associated issues.

They have been researched extensively, since its initial clinical trials began in the 1960s, Beta-blockers have been used for many years. As a result, their actions are more clearly known, making it simpler to utilise them properly and prevent side effects.

Because beta-blockers are frequently quite inexpensive, it is easier for patients to buy.

Risks: Beta-blockers can cause a variety of negative effects since they have an impact on your heart and circulatory systems. As a result, doctors frequently recommend particular beta-blockers to reduce or prevent these negative effects.

The following are typical negative effects of beta-blockers:

- Sluggish heartbeat (bradycardia).
- Reduced blood pressure (hypotension).
- Abnormal heartbeats (arrhythmia).
- Fatigue.
- Dizziness.
- Nausea.
- Nightmares, disturbed sleep, and insomnia.
- Dry eyes or mouth.
- Erectile and sexual dysfunction.

Beta-blockers may have a deleterious effect on several illnesses, ailments, and health issues. The following are examples of contraindications:

Severe to very serious asthma: Nonselective beta-blockers have the potential to exacerbate asthma attacks or induce breathing difficulties. For patients with less severe respiratory issues, doctors will frequently prescribe B1-selective beta-blockers to reduce this, but they will not use beta-blockers at all for patients with moderate to severe issues.
A few specific arrhythmias: Certain arrhythmias can be made worse by beta-blockers.
Low blood pressure or a slow heartbeat: By further reducing heart rate and blood pressure, the majority of beta-blockers will exacerbate either of these problems.
Raynaud's syndrome: Your hands, feet, particularly your fingers, and toes, and occasionally even some areas of your face, experience impaired circulation as a result of this illness. Beta-blockers could make the situation worse. Primary Raynaud's, sometimes referred to as Raynaud's syndrome or Raynaud's disease can happen on its own or as a result of another illness (secondary Raynaud's).
Hypoglycemia (low blood sugar): Beta-blockers help postpone the majority of low blood sugar's effects. This can delay taking action to regulate blood sugar levels for those with illnesses like diabetes (particularly Type 1) that produce low

blood sugar. If the levels go too low, you could have confusion, fainting, or seizures. Sweating is a significant sign of low blood sugar that beta-blockers do not cover-up. Those who use beta-blockers and are at risk of having low blood sugar should be aware of sudden perspiration as a warning indication.

If your symptoms, especially those that affect your heart and circulatory system, suddenly change, see a doctor. They consist of:

- Respiration difficulty.
- Ache in the chest.
- Heart flutters (where you can feel your heartbeat racing, pounding, or skipping beats).
- Suddenly passing out, or experiencing repeated Episodes of dizziness or lightheadedness.

Additional signs and symptoms to be aware of and discuss with your doctor include:

- Slow heartbeat, low blood pressure, confusion, or changes in behaviour, especially when they occur simultaneously. A beta-blocker overdose may be indicated by this cluster of symptoms. Beta-blockers can be used for a long time. In some circumstances, particularly for persons over 65, they may be used for years or permanently.

Nitrates

Nitrates are drugs that are used to treat or prevent angina, or chest discomfort, which is a symptom of heart disease and typically affects the arteries in the heart.

Nitrates are vasodilators, which expand the diameter of blood vessels to facilitate easier blood flow. The heart must work against the strong blood pressure in the arteries to pump blood from the body's veins back into the arteries through the lungs. The heart's muscle must generate and utilise energy (or "fuel") to complete its work, and this necessitates consuming oxygen that is provided by the blood. An inadequate supply of blood and oxygen to the heart muscle and causes angina (also known as angina pectoris, or "heart agony").

By dilating (expanding) the arteries and veins in the body, nitrates, such as isosorbide dinitrate, improve the flow of blood and oxygen to the heart and so enhance the work that the heart can perform.

Negative effects include:

- Kidney injury (this is rare).

- Birth defects
- Hyperkalemia (high blood potassium)
- Kidney disease.
- Low blood pressure.
- Stillbirth.

Your healthcare provider will prescribe a different medication that is safe for both you and your unborn child if you already have high blood pressure before becoming pregnant or if you acquire it whilst pregnant (preeclampsia). Always consult your healthcare professional before taking over-the-counter medications or supplements if you are taking blood pressure medication. Nonsteroidal anti-inflammatory drugs (NSAIDs) and several medications for colds, coughs, and allergies might raise blood pressure. This counteracts the effects of the ARBs

Calcium Channels Blockers

A class of drugs known as calcium channel blockers control how much calcium your body can use. These drugs can lower your blood pressure, avoid cardiac rhythm issues, and do other things by slowing down how your cells use calcium. There are two primary categories of calcium channel blockers. They are

- Dihydropyridines. They are particularly helpful at treating high blood pressure because they target blood arteries and encourage their relaxation.
- Non-dihydropyridines. These drugs effectively address issues with cardiac rhythm because they target both the heart muscle and the blood arteries.

As calcium is an electrolyte, when it dissolves in water, it acquires a positive charge. Ions (atoms with an electrical charge) in electrolytes are used by your body to transfer substances into and out of your cells. Your body is always trying to keep balance. This suggests that sodium ions leave a cell when calcium ions enter, and vice versa.

These ions enter and leave your cells through channels, which function similarly to doors leading within your cells. Also, those channels have a safety mechanism that restricts ion entry and exit to those with the proper size and kind of charge (either positive or negative).

Calcium channel blockers benefit from the fact that particular kinds of calcium channels frequently only exist in specific regions of the body. As a result, drugs can be targeted according to the channels they affect.

Every one of the cells in question has a large number of calcium channels. Calcium channel blockers, also known as calcium channel antagonists, only completely block some of them when used in the proper dosage. As a result, those cells consume calcium more slowly since there are fewer pathways for calcium to enter them.

- Diseases treated by calcium channel blockers
- Elevated blood pressure (hypertension).
- Arrhythmia (irregular heartbeat rhythms).
- Chest discomfort (angina).
- Heart muscle spasm.
- Hypertrophic Cardiomyopathy (enlarged heart).
- Hypertension in the lungs.
- Subarachnoid bleeding (bleeding into the space between the brain and the skull).

RISKS AND Benefits

Calcium channel blockers are frequently prescribed due to their many benefits.

These work well. People of all ages and races can benefit from calcium channel blockers, which are beneficial in treating a variety of associated cardiac and circulation issues.

They can target particular diseases. Different effects are more likely to occur based on the type of medication taken.

They might be a superior choice. Many drugs can lower blood pressure, however, some are not recommended for everyone. It may occur as a result of their current drugs, other medical illnesses they may have, their lifestyle, and other factors. A calcium channel blocker is a superior option for treatment in those circumstances.

They may function in conjunction with other drugs. Several medications, particularly those that treat problems like excessive cholesterol, mix calcium channel blockers with other pharmaceuticals. Many find it simpler to take their drugs while receiving combined therapy, which simultaneously addresses several issues.

Risks: The most frequent negative effects of dihydropyridines are:

- Feeling faint or disoriented.
- Having a flush.
- Headaches.
- Swelling limbs

Non-dihydropyridines, these drugs are likely to cause:

- Constipation.
- Sluggish heartbeat (bradycardia).
- Decreased capacity of your heart to pump blood.

Many calcium channel blockers might result in gingival hyperplasia, a condition in which the gums around your teeth swell excessively. The signs of gastroesophageal reflux disease (GERD) or heartburn may also worsen as a result of them.

Those with specific heart conditions or low blood pressure may not be able to take calcium channel blockers in general. Pregnancy, heart conditions, liver issues, or specific forms of abnormal heart rhythms are some other factors that may prevent you from using some of these medications.

If you have any of the following symptoms when taking Calcium channel blockers, see your doctor:

- Respiration difficulty.
- Pain in the chest, especially rapid shifts in its frequency or intensity.
- Irregular heartbeats (arrhythmia) or palpitations in the heart (where you can feel your heartbeat racing, pounding, or skipping beats).
- Abruptly fainting or experiencing frequent episodes of lightheadedness or vertigo.

- Moderate to severe rash or skin irritation without apparent cause.
- Swelling of the limbs, legs, or face, particularly around the eyes, lips, and tongue.

Diuretics

Diuretics, commonly referred to as water pills, are medications that aid in eliminating excess fluid and salt from the body. It should be taken before anything else in the morning if you can because they cause you to urinate more frequently. Diuretics may be required once or twice a day and at the exact time every day. Your kidneys are forced to excrete more water and salt as a result.

Diuretics are necessary for people with high blood pressure or excessive fluid retention.

Diuretics lower blood pressure by assisting your blood vessels in expanding. Also, there is less fluid in your blood for your heart to pump. Diuretics also assist your body in eliminating surplus fluids. Diuretics are typically taken as pills, but while you are in the hospital, your doctor may provide some of them through an IV in your arm. Most people can use diuretics without experiencing any major side effects. Diuretics treat:

- Heart attack.

- Cardiomyopathy.
- Pulmonary edema.
- Ascites.
- Renal dysfunction.
- Nephrotic syndrome
- Type 2 diabetes.
- An elevated intraocular pressure.
- High pressure inside the skull.

Benefits: Even older folks see positive effects from diuretics, especially when used to treat high blood pressure. Moreover, most people do not experience negative side effects from diuretics.
- Diuretic side effects frequently include:
- Increased urination.
- Dizziness.
- Tiredness.
- Headache.
- Gout.
- Erectile dysfunction
- Low potassium (unless you are using a diuretic kind that spares potassium).
- Muscle pain.
- A racing heart.
- Elevated blood sugar levels in diabetics.
- Dehydration.

- An electrolyte imbalance.

Your provider will want to check to be sure your kidneys are performing well and your potassium level is appropriate when you are taking diuretic medicines. Talk to your doctor about the dangers of diuretics if you are pregnant, breastfeeding, an older adult, or have kidney or liver issues.

Discuss the duration of your pharmaceutical regimen with your doctor. Never discontinue using these drugs without first consulting your doctor.

Surgeries For Heart Disease Treatment

Coronary Angioplasty And Stents

The treatment known as percutaneous coronary intervention, commonly known as coronary angioplasty, is performed to clear blocked heart arteries. A tiny balloon catheter is placed during an angioplasty procedure to assist widen a blood artery that has become narrowed and enhance blood flow to the heart.

A thin wire gauze tube known as a stent is always inserted in addition to an angioplasty. The stent assists in keeping the artery open, reducing the likelihood of further narrowing. To keep the artery open, medicine is usually coated on the most part of stents (drug-eluting stents). Bare-metal stents are used infrequently.

Chest pain and constantly being out of breath are examples of symptoms of blocked arteries that can be improved by an angioplasty. Angioplasty is often done to unblock a clogged artery immediately during a heart attack to lessen the amount of damage to the heart.

You may benefit from angioplasty as a form of treatment if:

- You have tried many drugs and lifestyle modifications, but nothing has helped your heart health.
- Your angina (chest pain) is getting worse.
- Your heart stops beating.

Risks: Although bypass surgery is a more invasive method of opening blocked arteries, angioplasty still entails significant hazards.

The most typical angioplasty risks are as follows:

- Your artery needs to be re-narrowed: There is a slight possibility that the treated artery will reoccur with angioplasty and drug-eluting stent implantation. The use of bare-metal

stents increases the chance of the artery re-
narrowing.

- Clotting of blood: Stents are susceptible to
blood clot formation even after the surgery.
These clots can seal the artery, triggering a
heart attack. To lessen the possibility of
blood clots forming in your stent, it is crucial
to take aspirin together with clopidogrel
(Plavix), prasugrel (Effient), or another drug
precisely as directed.
- Bleeding. When a catheter is implanted in
your leg or arm, there may be bleeding. Most
of the time, this just causes a bruise, but
occasionally, significant bleeding happens
and may need surgery or a blood transfusion.

The following are rare dangers angioplasty:

- Chest pains: Although extremely
unlikely, you could get a heart attack
while having the surgery.

Arterial damage in the heart: During the surgery,
the coronary artery could be ripped or ruptured.
These issues might necessitate urgent bypass
surgery.

- Kidney issues: Your doctor may take
precautions to try to protect your kidneys if
you are at an elevated risk, such as decreasing

the amount of contrast dye and making sure
you are well-hydrated throughout the
procedure.

- Stroke: If plaques come loose while the
catheters are being put through the aorta
during angioplasty, a stroke could result.
Moreover, blood clots can develop in
catheters and, should they come loose, go to
the brain. Stroke is a very uncommon side
effect of coronary angioplasty. To lower the
danger, blood thinners are given during the
surgery.

- Irregular heartbeats. The heart could beat too
quickly or too slowly during the process.
Although these heart rhythm issues are often
transient, sometimes medicine or a transient
pacemaker is required.

Cardiovascular Stent

The majority of patients who undergo angioplasty
also have a stent inserted into their blocked artery at
the same time. After angioplasty, a stent, which
resembles a tiny coil of wire mesh, supports the
walls of your artery and aids in preventing it from
re-narrowing. To keep the artery open and increase
blood flow to your heart, the stent remains in place

forever. To clear a blockage, more than one stent may occasionally be required. The balloon catheter is inflated and removed after the stent has been positioned.

Additional X-ray images are obtained (angiograms) to examine the blood flow via your enlarged artery. The majority of stents placed during an angioplasty are coated with drugs. The medication in the stent is progressively released to assist prevent future plaque formation and the re-narrowing of the blood channel.

Call your doctor immediately if:

- You have pain or discomfort where your catheter was placed.
- You exhibit symptoms of infection, such as fever, redness, edema, or discharge.
- The arm or limb that underwent the treatment has changed in warmth or colour.
- You feel weak or dizzy.
- You have shortness of breath or chest pain

Coronary Bypass Graft

A procedure used to treat coronary artery disease is coronary artery bypass graft surgery (CABG). The blood channels that carry oxygen and nutrients to the heart muscle are known as the coronary arteries, and coronary artery disease (CAD) is the narrowing of these blood vessels. Fatty substance accumulating in the artery walls is what leads to CAD. This accumulation makes the inside of the arteries smaller, which reduces the amount of oxygen-rich blood that can reach the heart muscle.

Bypassing the blocked section of the coronary artery with a piece of a healthy blood vessel from another part of your body is one method of treating the blocked or restricted arteries. Pieces of a leg vein or a chest artery may be utilised as blood arteries, or grafts, during the bypass treatment. Another option is to use an artery from your wrist. The graft is attached with one end above the blockage and the other below the blockage by your doctor. To get to the heart muscle, blood travels through the new graft and around the obstruction.

Your doctor typically creates a significant chest incision to bypass the blocked coronary artery while also momentarily stopping the heart. Your doctor will split the breastbone (sternum), which opens the chest, in half lengthwise, exposing the heart, and inserts tubes so that a heart-lung bypass machine can pump blood across the body once it has been exposed. This is done by stopping the heart from beating. Even though you might not experience any symptoms in the early stages of coronary artery disease, the condition will worsen until there is enough arterial blockage to result in symptoms and issues. You could experience a heart attack if the blood flow to your heart muscle keeps getting worse due to a coronary artery that is becoming increasingly blocked. The tissue of the heart muscle dies if the blood flow cannot be restored to the specific place that is injured.

Your doctor may advise CABG surgery for additional factors.

If you experience any of the following after the procedure, let your doctor know:

- A fever of at least 100.4°F (38°C), or chills
- Any signs of inflammation, edema, bleeding, or fluid from the incision sites
- Worsening of the discomfort at any of the incision locations
- Difficulty in breathing
- Quick or irregular heartbeat
- Swelling and numbness of arms and legs
- Persistent dizziness or nausea

Heart Transplant

A heart transplant is a surgical procedure where the patient's unhealthy heart is removed and replaced with a healthy heart from an organ donor. Two or more medical professionals must certify the donor as brain dead before the heart can be removed. A condition known as end-stage heart failure occurs when the heart muscle fails miserably to pump blood throughout the body. It denotes the failure of alternative treatments. A healthcare professional must determine that a heart transplant is the best course of treatment for your heart failure before you may be placed on a waiting list for one. It must also be established that you are in overall good health before the transplant. Your doctor might suggest a heart transplant for additional causes.

What dangers come with a heart transplant? Difficulties can arise during surgery. The following are possible dangers of a heart transplant:

- Infection
- Bleeding during or following the procedure
- Clots in the blood that can result in heart attack, stroke, or lung issues
- Breathing difficulties
- Renal failure
- Death
- Donor heart failure
- Poor circulation of blood Throughout the body, including the brain.

- Serious medical conditions, other than the heart disease, would not improve after the transplant

Consult your doctor if you experience:

- Either a fever or chills. This could indicate infection or rejection.
- The incision site or any of the catheter sites are red, swollen, or bleeding.
- Increased discomfort near the site of the incision
- Difficulty in breathing
- Excessive tiredness
- Reduced blood pressure

Depending on your particular situation, your healthcare professional might offer you additional advice after the treatment.

You will require lifelong medication to prevent rejection for the transplanted heart to survive in your body. Drug reactions might vary from person to person, and adverse effects can be severe. To match your needs, your healthcare professional will customise your medication.

CHAPTER 6

HEART HEALTH AND NUTRITION

The best diet for preventing heart disease includes plenty of fruits and vegetables, whole grains, nuts, fish, poultry, and vegetable oils. It also includes alcohol, you can drink in moderation and limit red and processed meats, refined carbohydrates, foods, and drinks with added sugar, sodium, and trans fats. A diet heavy in cholesterol, trans fats, and saturated fats has been associated with atherosclerosis and other illnesses like heart disease. Also, too much salt (sodium) intake can cause blood pressure to rise. If you drink, a small glass of red wine can be a heart-healthy option. Red wine contains two antioxidants, resveratrol and catechins, which may shield arterial walls.The good cholesterol HDL can also be increased by alcohol. Alcohol abuse damages the heart. Never consume more than one drink for ladies or two for men each day. It is best to first speak with your doctor. Those who use aspirin and other drugs may experience issues after consuming alcohol.

Foods That May Save Your Heart

Fresh Herbs: Making the decision to add these to food in place of salt and fat is heart-healthy. They enhance flavour without the undesirables. Delicious methods to eat heart-smartly is to include spices with other foods.

Black beans: Black beans are mild, delicate, and full of minerals that are good for the heart. Blood pressure can be lowered with magnesium, folate, and antioxidants. Their fibre aids in blood sugar and cholesterol regulation. To improve soups and salads, add beans.

Salmon: It is a top food for heart health because it is omega-3-rich. Healthy fats called omega-3s may lower blood pressure and reduce the risk of heart rhythm problems. They might also reduce inflammation and triglycerides. Two meals with salmon or other oily fish per week are advised by the American Heart Association.

Tuna: Tuna has omega-3s and is frequently less expensive than salmon. In comparison to other tuna varieties, albacore (white tuna) contains greater omega-3s. Try grilling tuna steak with lemon and dill. Add mackerel, herring, lake trout, sardines, and anchovies as additional omega-3 sources.

Olive oil: Made from crushed olives, this oil is a good source of fat. Antioxidants that promote heart health are abundant. Your blood vessels might be protected by using Olive oil. It can reduce cholesterol levels when it is used in place of saturated fats like butter. Serve it with toast, cooked vegetables, and salads.

Walnuts: A daily serving of a few walnuts may help decrease cholesterol and might also shield your arteries from being inflamed. Omega-3 fatty acids, monounsaturated fats, plant sterols, and fibre are all abundant in walnuts. The advantages occur when walnuts replace unhealthy fats, such as those found in cookies and chips.

Almonds: With vegetables, fish, fowl, and desserts, slivered almonds pair well. Almonds consist of fibre, heart-healthy lipids, and plant sterols. The consumption of almonds may reduce "bad" LDL cholesterol. Every day, take a little handful.

Sweet potatoes: Eat sweet potatoes in place of white potatoes. Compared to white potatoes, these potatoes have a lower glycemic index, therefore they will not induce a sharp rise in blood sugar. They are also rich in lycopene, fibre, and vitamin A.

Oranges: Oranges are sweet and juicy, and they include the cholesterol-lowering fibre, pectin and potassium, which aids in blood pressure regulation. Two cups of orange juice per day will improve blood vessel health.

Swiss Chard: This leafy dark green vegetable is high in magnesium and potassium. These minerals aid in blood pressure regulation. Furthermore, heart-healthy fibre, vitamin A, and the antioxidants lutein and zeaxanthin are all present in Swiss chard. Use it with grilled meats or use it to serve on fish.

Barley: Try substituting this nutty whole grain for rice. Barley can be used to cook stews and soups. Barley's dietary fibre can reduce cholesterol levels. It could also reduce blood sugar levels.

Oatmeal: Oatmeal is beneficial for diabetics as well since it keeps blood sugar levels consistent over time, fills you up for hours, and prevents snack attacks. Fibre oats lower harmful cholesterol, which is good for your heart. Oats are best cooked on a low heat.

Flaxseed: Three components of this glossy, honey-coloured seed fibre, lignan-related phytonutrients, and omega-3 fatty acids are heart-healthy.

Fat-Free Yogurt: You probably think, "Excellent for my bones!" when you think about dairy foods. Moreover, these foods can lower blood pressure. Potassium and calcium levels in yoghurt are high.

Choose low-fat options to effectively increase the calcium content while reducing the fat.

Sterols fortified foods: Sterols and stanols, which lower cholesterol, are added to some types of margarine, soy milk, almond milk, and orange juice. These plant extracts prevent the absorption of cholesterol by your stomach. They can reduce LDL levels by 10% without affecting HDL.

Cherries: Cherry juice, dried cherries, sweet cherries, and sour cherries are all delectable. They are loaded with antioxidants. All are rich in anthocyanins, an antioxidant. They may aid in blood vessel defence.

Blueberries: Just brilliant in terms of nutrition is blueberries. They contain antioxidants called anthocyanins, that support blood vessels and also give the berries it's colour. Moreover, blueberries contain fibre and a wide range of other beneficial elements. Add them either fresh or dried, to your yoghurt, pancakes, or cereal.

Dark Green Leaves: When your parents advised you to eat your greens, they were on to something. They are rich in minerals and vitamins and contain a lot of nitrates too, which helps to widen blood vessels so that oxygen-rich blood can flow to your heart. They are present in vegetables and greens such as lettuce, Spinach, Bok Choy, Mustard, and Arugula

Supplements And Nutrients That Promote Heart Health

Fibre: Cereals made of oats and bran are a heart-healthy way to start the day. The soluble fibre included in them aids in reducing LDL "bad" cholesterol.

Beans and healthy grains like barley are additional excellent sources. Like psyllium, you can also purchase it as a supplement, but a diet high in fibre is the best

.

Stanols And Sterols: These nutrients can be found in a few fruits, vegetables, nuts, and seeds. They prevent cholesterol from being absorbed by your body. Good options include almonds, peanuts, olive oil, and Brussels sprouts.

Moreover, keep an eye out for foods like yoghurt, margarine, and orange juice that have sterols and stanols added to them. Supplements may help lower your cholesterol, but see your doctor first.

Garlic: You might also safeguard your heart when you spice up your food. Garlic has been used as medicine for centuries, and studies on dietary supplements suggest it may lower cholesterol and blood pressure. Before taking any tablets, consult your doctor first as they may increase your risk of bleeding and conflict with other medications you are taking.

Vitamin D: There are hardly many meals that contain it, yet it helps to keep your heart healthy. Some of them include tuna and salmon. Moreover, it is present in vitamin D-fortified milk and orange juice. Its applications and the potential benefit of supplements are still being researched. If your doctor advises it, take them.

The fatty acids omega-3: They aid in maintaining healthy arteries, maintaining stable blood pressure, and lowering triglycerides, which are blood lipids that can increase your risk of heart disease. Consuming fish with lots of fat like salmon or mackerel twice a week is a wonderful method to get this nutrient. Try fish oil tablets if your doctor thinks you need to consume extra omega-3s, but be sure to inquire about the recommended dosage.

Catechins: To reduce your risk of heart disease and stroke, drink green tea. Catechins, which are compounds found in it, may lower your cholesterol, according to research. Ask your doctor before taking

the capsule version if you do not like the taste of this
beverage.

Lycopene: Eating tomatoes, whether raw or cooked
in a sauce, will provide you with this chemical.
Although it is unclear how it functions, studies
indicate it reduces your risk of heart disease. You
can purchase it as a supplement, but researchers
think eating foods that naturally contain it is
preferable. The tomato's vitamin K promotes
circulation and controls bleeding and blood clotting.

Pectin: This kind of soluble fibre is present in fruits
like apples and strawberries, which lowers LDL
cholesterol. Health professionals advise eating it
naturally rather than taking a supplement, though
you can.

Soy: Adjust your diet and include items made from
this pea family plant. Tofu, soy milk, and edamame
are a few options. If you consume them instead of
meat that is high in fat, they will be beneficial for
your heart

Pomegranate: Strong antioxidants found in this
fruit can help keep your arteries clear and safeguard
your heart. While some people adore its tart flavour,
if you prefer something else and wish to take a

supplement, consult your doctor first. Certain medications can not mix well with supplements.

Folate: By eating meals high in this nutrient, you may lower your risk of heart attack and heart disease. You have a wide range of options. Eat lentils, lima beans, and asparagus, as well as dark leafy greens like spinach. Although it is available as a supplement, the American Heart Association advises eating a diet high in folate-rich foods.

CHAPTER 7

THE STATE OF ONE'S MIND AND EMOTIONS AS IT RELATES TO HEART'S HEALTH

Preventing and managing cardiac health includes taking good care of your mental health and wellness. It has been established that your heart's health and mental well-being are tightly related. Your cardiovascular health can be affected negatively by stress, despair, anxiety, rage, and social isolation. The following warning signals are provided to reassure you that you may have a valid reason to seek further information regarding your worries and to assist you in making a mental health issue diagnosis.

- Having fear or anxiety

Everybody experiences anxiety or tension from time to time. Yet, anxiety might not indicate a mental health issue. But, if anxiety persists and interferes constantly, it may be a symptom of a mental health issue. Additional signs of anxiety may include heart palpitations, shortness of breath, headache, sweating, shaking, feeling dizzy, restlessness, diarrhoea, or racing thoughts.

- Feeling down or unhappy

Being melancholy or angry for a few weeks or longer, missing energy and ambition, losing interest in a pastime, or crying constantly are all indications of depression.

- Mood swings

Everybody has varied emotions, but abrupt and drastic changes in mood, like acute distress or rage, might be a sign of mental illness.

- Issues with sleep

A mental health issue may show symptoms, including persistent alterations in sleep patterns. For instance, insomnia might be an indication of anxiety or drug usage. Oversleeping or undersleeping could be signs of depression or a sleeping condition.

- Changes in weight or appetite

Rapid weight loss or fluctuating weight may be one of the warning indicators of a mental health condition, such as depression or an eating disorder, for certain people.

- Reserved or reclusive

A mental health condition may be indicated if a person withdraws from life, especially if this is a significant change. If a friend or loved one is constantly isolated from everyone, they might be suffering from depression, bipolar disorder, a psychotic disorder, or another mental illness. They may need assistance if they decline to participate in social activities.

- Misuse of drugs

Alcohol or drug use as a coping mechanism might be an indication of mental health issues. Substance abuse might also aggravate the mental disease.

- Guilt or worthlessness

It is possible that thoughts like "I am a failure," "It is my fault," or "I am useless" are symptoms of a mental health issue like depression. If your friend or loved one is constantly criticising or blaming themselves, they could need help. A person may express the desire to harm or kill themself when it is serious. This emotion may indicate suicidal tendencies and the need for immediate assistance.

Modifications In Attitude Or Behaviour

A mental health illness may begin as minor adjustments to a person's emotions, thoughts, or behaviour. When these changes become frequent and serious it could indicate the mental health condition is on the horizon. It is crucial to start the dialogue about seeking assistance if something does not seem "quite right".

There are straightforward techniques to encourage mental wellness and lessen stress, which will aid you in managing your heart health as well. These are,

- Routine exercise
- Engaging in mindfulness
- Establishing connections to others to combat social Isolation
- Seeking expert guidance for mental health

How Might Exercise Enhance You Physical And Mental Health?

There is evidence that regular exercise lowers stress and improves mental health. You might be surprised to learn that after you start moving, you may feel more self-assured, sleep better, enjoy a decrease in depression and anxiety symptoms, and have the stamina to participate in more social interactions and activities.

The key to beginning and maintaining regular physical activity is finding a hobby or pastime that can fit into your daily routine. A few examples of physical activity are taking regular strolls, biking, swimming, dancing, practising yoga, playing golf, lifting weights, or participating in seasonal activities like snowshoeing or paddle boarding.

How Does Practising Mindfulness Help You To Feel Better Mentally?

By lowering stress, enhancing sleep, and making you feel more balanced and connected, practising mindfulness is another strategy to support mental wellness. There is emerging evidence, according to the British Heart Foundation, that practising mindfulness may help lower the risk of developing heart disease and stroke. As a fundamental human ability, mindfulness is the capacity to be fully present, and aware of where we are and what we are doing, without becoming unduly reactive or overwhelmed by what is happening around us. Through meditation, physical relaxation exercises, and breathing exercises, one can practise mindfulness.

In what ways does lowering social isolation lower your risk of heart disease?
Loneliness and social isolation have been associated with an increased risk of coronary heart disease. By lowering chronic stress and harmful coping mechanisms, which are frequently linked to

loneliness. Meaningful social contact, and support can protect the heart. You can try the following if you want to lessen social isolation and expand your social support network:

- Creating a new pastime
- Participating in community services
- Joining a neighbourhood or community group
- Joining a hiking, gardening, or book club
- Taking a course to acquire a new skill
- Joining a sports team or an exercise class

When Should You Get Help From A Professional To Keep Your Mental Health?

It might be time to seek professional guidance and assistance if stress management continues to be difficult for you or if you show signs of depression, anxiety, or both. To start, you can talk about stress management techniques with your family doctor or arrange a meeting with a local councillor.

The term "psychotherapist" refers to many distinct types of mental health specialists. Among them are therapists and psychologists. Each of these experts offers psychotherapy. A form of "talking treatment" is psychotherapy. Your emotional and physical well-being will be enhanced by it. The schools of psychotherapy are very diverse. These can include

expressive therapy, group therapy, and other
therapies as well as therapeutic talks. Cognitive
behavioural therapy is the most common type
(CBT). You can learn how to alter negative habits,
cognitive patterns, or emotions with the use of CBT.
Never stigmatise somebody for seeking help;

How Does The State Of One's Heart Depend On Their Emotions?

Your state of well-being ties to all aspects of your
life, including your emotional, social, spiritual,
physical, and intellectual well-being
Consider the condition known as stress
cardiomyopathy or shattered heart syndrome.
Research has found that within 24 hours of losing a
loved one, the chance of having a heart attack jumps
21-fold. In addition to the loss of a loved one, the
heart can also be damaged by other shocks. A loved
one being diagnosed with cancer, for example,
might trigger stress cardiomyopathy. Strong feelings
like rage can also lead to irregular heartbeats. Your
heart might also suffer from stress. Your blood
pressure and heart rate increase while you are under
stress. Your body is subjected to unhealthily high
levels of stress chemicals like cortisol from chronic
stress, which can alter the way blood clots. A heart

attack or stroke may be precipitated by any of these elements. For instance, individuals who experience chronic stress, anxiety, depression, or anger may be more prone to unhealthy habits that are harmful to their hearts, such as excessive alcohol consumption, smoking, overeating, and inactivity.

What Happens If Your Heart Is Already Weak?
A crucial component of total health is emotional well-being. Emotional stress can worsen cardiac disease, which already exists. Patients with anxiety who have heart disease are twice as likely to pass away within three years of a cardiac incident. Furthermore, depression is three times more common in people with cardiac problems. Depression increases the likelihood that a dangerous heart-related event may occur within a year for people who have just received a heart disease diagnosis. Major depression doubles the risk of dying from heart-related causes even in those without prior heart disease, so the American Heart Association advises that every cardiac patient must undergo routine depression screening. The demands of cardiac patients' mental health are also a focus of the new emotion-based approach to heart health known as cardiac psychology. It advocates using

techniques to assist people to deal with their illness,
such as stress reduction and psychotherapy.
Heart and mind are in harmony. Do not dismiss
feelings like ongoing tension, worry, despair, or rage
that have the potential to take over your life. Your
heart will reward you if you find strategies to take
care of your emotional well-being.
Feelings should be acknowledged and expressed.
Join a support group, or speak with loved ones.
Request for professional assistance if the need
arises. Do deep breathing techniques, yoga, or daily
mindful meditation to reduce stress. Do not drink
too much alcohol and do not smoke.
Exercise, consider going for a quick 15-minute
stroll, swimming, cycling, gardening, or dancing.
Have a nutritious diet that is high in omega-3 fatty
acids because they have anti-inflammatory
properties.

When you are aware of the emotions that make you
not feel good and communicate them to yourself and
others in a positive way, your resilience increases.
The people closest to you, your family, your
neighbours, your coworkers, and, inevitably, the
most defenceless, your children will almost certainly

receive your anguish if you do not alter it. Start by noticing and controlling your thoughts, feelings, and behaviours if you want to overcome that challenge. It influences your course of action and fundamentally alters how you respond to pressure-filled circumstances and make judgments. As your emotional health becomes more important to you, you become better equipped to Provide and accept feedback from a perspective that is healthy, conduct uncomfortable conversations and discussions with anyone, and build stronger connections.

What Are Some Examples of Emotional Well-Being?

You will be better able to deal with situations that may or may not be beyond your control if you have strong emotional health. You might utilise one of these techniques to get into a mindset that enables you to control your emotions when confronted with a difficult scenario.

Breathe, centre yourself, and take a moment.

This straightforward three-step procedure can aid you in gaining better emotional control during a difficult scenario.

- Take a breath. When you breathe deeply, your brain receives a signal that promotes relaxation and calmness.
- Remain rooted. Possess a pen. Seize a desk's edge. Feel the ground beneath your feet. You leave your difficult thoughts behind and return to the present.
- Pause, and wait. afterward, ask yourself, "What do I want to say?" You are in a condition of emotional well-being when you have the words to say what you need to say.

Your emotional health is influenced by your range of emotions and how you handle them. These are some strategies for maintaining emotional control and resilience:

Activate your body: Engage in some type of physical activity. Exercise. Dance. Organise laundry. If the weather is suitable, go outside.

Create a routine: Schedule your meetings accordingly. Set aside time to set goals. Make space for reading. Prepare a fresh meal. Take a musical break.

Get in touch with others: Do your family a favour. Contact the people that are behind you. Enquire about assistance. Be brave to leave your comfort zone, and learn something new. Be with someone you respect and spend quality time together.

Forgive: When you forgive, you should also forgive yourself. You can retain your authority when you forgive. Living in the present moment is made possible by forgiveness. Growth and happiness are also made possible by forgiveness.

Sleep: Your body has an opportunity to heal itself during sound sleep. Your memory and information-processing skills improve when you get enough sleep. You feel happier when you awaken.

Kindly ask yourself, What makes you happy? Where do you feel most calm? When will you feel free to be yourself? When you are good to yourself, you will want to be kind to others as well. Know yourself: Take note of your positive ideas, deeds, routines, and character traits. Also, you will be ready and aware of the changes that need to be made when you see them. Emotionally balanced people have control over their ideas, feelings, and actions. They can handle the difficulties of life and are capable of remaining optimistic and bounce back from failures. They have positive self-esteem and satisfying relationships. Being emotionally stable does not necessarily entail constant joy. It means that you are aware of your feelings and what goes on around you. No matter how they turn out, you can manage them. Pressure,anger, and sorrow are also felt by emotionally healthy persons. But they don't embrace their negative emotions. They can recognize when a situation is too much for them to tackle alone. Also,they know when to consult a doctor. Your ability to work efficiently and handle life's difficulties depends on your emotional well-being. You might be able to reach your maximum potential. It enables you to collaborate with others and give back to the community. Your physical health is also impacted. According to research, a positive outlook on life is associated with outward manifestations of health. They include a healthier weight, lower blood pressure, and a lower risk of heart disease.

Embracing Good Feelings

From love and gratitude to laughter and other pleasurable experiences, it has been demonstrated that these things significantly lower your risk of heart attack and stroke and may even lengthen your life. Compared to those who are pessimistic, those who are most optimistic are twice as likely to have perfect cardiovascular health.

The risk of heart attack and stroke is reduced by 50% in happy persons. A recent review found that, even after accounting for factors including age, socioeconomic level, smoking, and body weight, feelings of optimism, life satisfaction, and happiness were associated with a decreased risk for cardiovascular disease (CVD). The chance of an initial cardiovascular event, such as a heart attack or stroke, was just half as high for the most cheery individuals as it was for the least hopeful. A balanced diet, exercise, and adequate sleep are just a few examples of healthier practices that happy individuals exhibit. Together with lower blood pressure, better lipid profiles, and healthier body weight, an optimistic outlook was also linked to these factors. Our results indicate that strengthening psychological assets rather than only addressing psychological deficits may have a positive impact on cardiovascular health. An optimistic perspective might lessen inflammation. Even when potential confounders are taken into account, women who experience more positive emotions throughout a typical day are less likely to have high blood levels of the inflammatory biomarker high-sensitivity C-reactive protein (hsCRP) than women who experience few or no moments of joy. Another study, which included participants from various ethnic backgrounds, connected pessimism to higher levels of CRP and fibrinogen (a protein involved in blood clotting). More than a dozen significant studies have found that excessive levels of hs-CRP indicate a higher risk of heart disease, including a double or tripled risk for heart attacks, strokes, developing peripheral artery disease, and dying suddenly of cardiac causes.

Having fun may be as healthy for your blood vessels as exercising. Have a good belly laugh every day because watching comedies improve vascular function whereas watching sombre films has the reverse impact.

CHAPTER 8

ADJUSTING TO LIFE WITH HEART DISEASE

Living with a cardiac ailment may need you to accept what has happened and how it may have affected various facets of your life. Several sorts of emotional distress or behavioural disorder may occur. Anxiety and depression-related issues are particularly prevalent. These issues can have an impact on your heart disease symptoms in addition to how you feel emotionally. Thankfully, there are effective treatments for anxiety and depression, including psychotherapies like cognitive behaviour therapy (CBT) and antidepressant drugs. It will be more simple to adhere to your heart disease treatment plan if you take care of these issues. Your healthcare providers, such as your general practitioner or a cardiac rehabilitation nurse, will be able to assist in evaluating any worries you may have about your psychological health.

Rehabilitation For The Heart

After a heart attack, heart surgery, or other heart operations, many hospitals have a cardiac rehabilitation program administered by cardiac rehabilitation nurses and physiotherapists that will help you regain your fitness and confidence as well as give you information and advice. You might receive a visit from a member of the cardiac rehabilitation team who will inform you about your condition, your course of care, and progress.

A cardiac rehabilitation program should also extend an invitation to you, starting four to eight weeks after you leave the hospital. Rehab should be made available to you if you have had:

- A cardiac arrest
- Angioplasty of the heart
- An open heart operation
- Angina or cardiac arrest (for some people)
- An inserted ICD (for some people)

Some programs are held in a hospital or public space. These workshops will provide you and your family with the knowledge, encouragement, and guidance you need to return to regular life as quickly as possible.

Cardiac rehabilitation benefits you by:

Recognizing your condition

- Recuperating after your operation, procedure, or heart attack
- Alter your way of life to safeguard your heart
- Lessen the likelihood of new issues arising.

Keeping your cardiac condition under control

The nature of your continuous follow-up and review will change depending on your cardiac condition and personal circumstances. The frequency of your visits to your cardiologist may fluctuate over time, or you may see other medical specialists, such as your general practitioner. It is crucial to follow up with any check ups because they are an excellent tool to monitor your health generally, including your heart condition. You will also have your blood pressure and pulse checked, as well as your weight (and perhaps your waist) measured. Together with your lifestyle, symptoms, mental health, and wellness, questions will be asked of you. You will typically undergo annual blood tests, however, they can be more frequent later on, particularly after initial medication therapies.

Hospital Evaluations

Hospital evaluations will be scheduled as needed. In more specialised circumstances, an ECG (electrocardiogram) may be requested of you, and occasionally further examinations will also be conducted. You must continue with your medication. Some people may find this difficult, particularly if they have never had to take medication before. There are many different kinds of medicines that can be recommended. Despite the fact that they may appear identical, it is crucial that you only take your prescriptions and never stop them without consulting a doctor. You can ask your doctor for further details about your drugs in addition to discussing your situation with them.

Managing Oneself

A period of having a heart ailment may be brief for some people. Yet, it will alter how the majority of patients live their lives. If you have a cardiac issue, you might want to adjust your lifestyle in some significant or modest ways. An important component of such long-term management will be the support, care, and treatment provided by formal health and social care agencies. Yet, the patients will typically be taking care of their disease on their own, with assistance from family and friends. This is self-management.

Going back to work

After receiving a diagnosis of a heart ailment or heart disease, you might need to undergo cardiac rehabilitation before going back to work. This will primarily depend on the kind of work you do and the level of physical and mental activity required, such as manual labour or a desk job. Before going back to work, you might want to discuss your options with your employer, your medical team, and the occupational health department.

After receiving a diagnosis of a heart problem or disease, you and your family may find it beneficial to talk about any benefits and support you are entitled to if you are unable to return to your employment. Finding out you might no longer be able to perform your job can be stressful, therefore it is crucial to discuss this with your family or other close friends to help ease your fears and anxieties.

Relationships

After receiving a diagnosis of a heart ailment or heart disease, many people experience relationship anxiety. It may cause you to feel depressed and alter how you view yourself as a person, as well as your position in the family or at home. Connections with partners, as well as those with friends and family, can be crucial in helping the person living with heart disease.

Sexual Interactions

Any significant health issue may affect your sexual life. Being a heart patient is the same thing. This is a significant concern for everybody who has ever engaged in sexual activity. If you are concerned, talk to your spouse and a health professional. With a diagnosis of heart disease or another cardiac ailment, many people worry that sex is not safe. For the majority of people, having sex is risk-free and comparable to exercising your heart. It does not put the heart under any greater strain than other forms of moderate exercise. Making love elevates the heart rate roughly as much as ascending two flights of stairs if you consider sex to be physical exercise. Sex boosts blood pressure like any workout does, but only momentarily. After that, your blood pressure instantly drops. This brief rise in blood pressure is safe and usual.

Being near to your spouse and helping them in a close and supportive way may feel more like your previous relationship and is also very crucial if your sexual relationship has deteriorated before the heart attack.

Talk to your doctor if you have any physical issues, such as erectile dysfunction (impotence), that are preventing you from having a normal sexual life. No drug should be taken without consulting a doctor after a heart attack or if you have any heart disease.

Palliative Medicine

There are certain patients whose heart disease progresses despite therapies, similar to other long-term diseases, necessitating a distinct strategy for continuous care. Supportive and palliative care symptom control techniques may be required if symptoms are increasingly resistant to standard treatment.

Your healthcare provider may want to discuss your ongoing wishes for your heart management and your preferred location of treatment with you and your loved ones as chronic heart failure progresses. This could result in a personalised care plan for advanced care that reflects your preferences. This necessitates using a supportive palliative care strategy to enhance the quality of life for those with life-threatening illnesses and their families, to prevent and ease suffering. Identify, evaluate, and treat physical, psychological, and spiritual concerns including pain. Affirm life and view the process of dying as natural provide a network of assistance to enable patients to lead as active a life as possible.

CHAPTER 9

Techniques to enhance the quality of life

When someone is diagnosed with heart disease, they may experience worry, anxiety, and uncertainty. You can also have a lot of queries and worries about what will come next, from selecting a course of treatment to paying for it. Although there is no right or wrong way to deal with heart disease, there are steps to help you feel more in control of your situation.

Here are 10 suggestions to assist you in adjusting to your diagnosis and raising your quality of life:

- Take it slow.

Strive to deal with one problem and one moment at a time. Let your thoughts drift away from the unknowns or the heart disease and toward what you can manage. The worst-case scenarios should not be projected for the future. You can feel less exposed

and have more control by taking one modest move
at a time.

- Request assistance.
Share your feelings honestly with your family and
friends, and let them know how they can help.
Provide specific examples like doing research on
insurance issues, taking notes at doctor's
appointments while you are there, or just listening
when you want to discuss. Join an online community
of support to create a network of online helpers
among your friends and family.

- Keep in touch with your medical staff.
Before each session, make a list of the questions you
have and take the time you need to get them
answered. Ask for more time with your doctor if you
need it. There might be longer appointments
available. They need to talk to you. Inform them if
you are having problems with the adverse effects.

- Have appropriate control over your life.
Feeling in control of your life can be challenging if
you have cardiovascular disease. Develop a plan
with the help of your loved ones and medical team
that provides you as much control over your life as

you want and can bear while receiving treatment. Learning more about your treatment options and the possible side effects might help you to be in control.

- Recognize your emotions and express them. Negative emotions may be brought on by a diagnosis. Discover healthy outlets for your emotions, such as writing, speaking, exercising, or engaging in creative endeavours. If sadness or anxiety are bothering you, seeking professional help is advised. Do not be afraid to tell your medical staff about this so you can get professional help. See your doctor if you suspect that you could be suffering from depression or anxiety.

- Consult with others who have cardiovascular disease for support.

When people converse with others going through similar problems, they find solace and strength. They provide a secure environment for patients, survivors, and caregivers to talk about their personal experiences and inspire others by sharing their insights and coping mechanisms. Dealing with side effects, diet and well-being, caregiver assistance, and other topics are covered. A nearby support group is another way to meet people.

- Acquire relaxation skills.

A peaceful, in-control physical condition is referred to as relaxation. It may be necessary for you to understand how to master relaxation because it is not always simple. Take into account pastimes that relax you. That could involve doing something relaxing like cooking, reading, walking, or meditating. To be at ease and to appreciate the present is the aim.

- Pursue your interests.

After receiving a heart diagnosis, you are not required to put your interests and goals on hold. Consider the prior pursuits that gave your life joy and significance. Do you have any hobbies you have always wanted to try but have not yet? Consider engaging in those activities right away if you can do them comfortably and safely and your healthcare provider agrees. Your quality of life may be greatly improved by making time for your enjoyable activities.

- Adopt a healthy lifestyle.

Making changes to improve your well-being can always be done at any time. Establish attainable goals and progress toward them. Enhance your diet and add feel-good exercises to your daily regimen. Your doctor can make safe workout suggestions. Taking care of your sleep hygiene is essential for ensuring that you receive enough rest and sleep. These are all techniques to enhance both physical and mental well-being.

- Keep a positive outlook.

Hope is both desirable and logical. Even though your experience is challenging, you can still set modest goals and take enjoyment in everyday activities. By concentrating on the things and people that make you happy, you may change the way that hopes feels to you. Hope spreads quickly. Spend time and surround yourself with things that make you feel this way.

Conclusion

Due to the typical American diet's reliance on high-sodium, processed foods, and animal products, conditions like high blood pressure, high cholesterol, and heart disease are particularly prevalent among Americans. Most Americans unknowingly follow a diet that is slowly shortening their lifespan and negatively affecting their health and well-being. Unfortunately, patients are all too frequently advised to seek a quick but risky fix, such as a drug or a treatment, when these diets lead to someone in the doctor's office or the emergency department. The underlying food and lifestyle behaviors that cause and exacerbate heart issues cannot be addressed by medications or surgery. Doctors rarely advise these patients to drastically alter their diets and lives to get better results. Even when physicians do offer this advice, they hardly ever do it with the level of specificity required to enable patients to empower themselves with the knowledge they need to succeed. Irreparable cardiac conditions or defects affect only 1% of persons. The remaining 99 percent of people have the chance to safeguard their health and longevity. To achieve this, people should choose foods that offer the most nutrients per calorie to increase the nutrient density in their diet. Those who heed this advice will inevitably steer clear of the most hazardous items, such as meats and refined sweets, which have high-calorie counts but little nutrients. People will instead go toward vegetables, fruits, beans, nuts, and seeds if they are looking for the most nutrient-dense diets. Cardiac disease has the highest mortality rate in men and women. The fact that over half of Americans have one or more of the three main risk factors for this condition high blood pressure, high cholesterol, or a smoking habit is not unexpected. Yet making healthy decisions can lessen or even eliminate all of these factors. There is no need for heart disease to be inevitable. By taking action, the threat can be eliminated.

The fact that patients almost always can prevent premature death from heart disease should be welcome news. Yet, the difficulty of maintaining a diet deters the majority of individuals from adopting the necessary, life-saving modifications since it is so difficult. For starters, the survival instinct is rooted in the fact that the human brain is designed to crave and seek out nourishment. Overcoming that need results in mental tension, which many people may react to by reaching for food. A struggle for willpower is not the solution because of this self-perpetuating cycle. One psychologist at the University of Minnesota suggests, instead, making it more difficult for individuals to get unhealthy meals so they will not have to rely on their willpower to make the right decision.

Majority of people give up on their efforts to work out or eat healthily because they wait for results before altering their entire perspective on their objectives. In other words, logging daily workouts or eating one nutritious meal at a time is insufficient. Instead, people must be willing to either embrace a nutrient-rich diet or risk losing their life to a preventable cardiac illness to make a life-altering adjustment, such as the kind necessary to reverse or prevent heart disease.